Energy Hacks

Energy Hacks

Energy Hacks

15 Simple Practical Hacks to Fight Fatigue and Get More Energy All Day

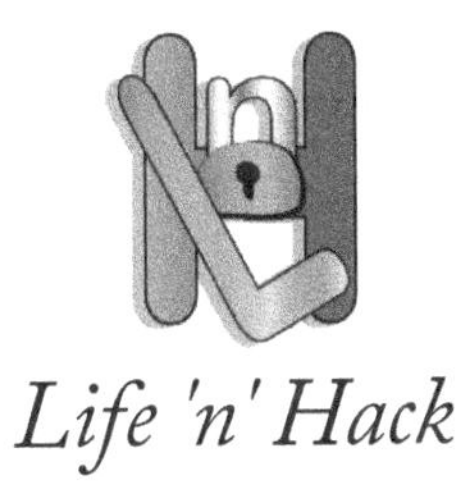

Life 'n' Hack

ISBN 978-1-976-37216-2

Printed in the United States of America

First Edition

KEYS

INFO UNLOCKED: Battery Fully Recharged

- 57 -

INFO INTRO:

Battery Running Low

We all know instinctively that our personal energy level determines how well we perform during the day, and to some extent all month long. Your energy not only feeds your body but is also the force behind your mental strength all during the day.

Take this scenario:

Let's say that you've just worked out and your body is in a lot of pain. Probably all you can think about is lying in bed and taking a snooze. Then, you suddenly remember you promised to rehearse a play with a friend right this instant. But you can't even muster the strength to move because all your energy has gone into that workout, and it won't come back until you've rested up—causing your body to shut down as well as your brain.

With that said, it's obvious that it's important to maintain and recharge your personal energy level instantly, manually, and efficiently.

Here are some reasons increasing your energy level can be beneficial for you:

- You have to get things done during the day, and if unexpected events that you didn't plan, predict, or prepare for come up, they will drain more of your energy. It's better to be ready than sorry.

- You need to face the demands of a very busy lifestyle because you understand the importance of working hard every day to make a living and support your family. That requires a consistent, sustainable amount of energy.

- You are tired all the time or experience chronic fatigue, it means your body is not rejuvenating itself properly. Something about your lifestyle, and possibly your diet, needs to change.

Besides these, working on building your personal energy is good for your overall health (body and nervous system).

Now, rather than tell you to stop doing the things that drain you (because some may even be a mandatory part of your daily life, such as your job), we suggest trying out the hacks that follow to help boost your energy and get you through your day with energy to spare.

Are you ready? Time to move on to our first energy-boosting hack on the list.

HACK #1:

Blast Icy Cold Showers

Have you ever watched a cartoon show where the hero gets energized after receiving an *electrical shock*? Well, that's a little like how this first hack works.

Do you know how people get when the shower ... suddenly turns cold? The shock of icy cold water makes them jump as if they were taken by surprise or wakened suddenly from a deep sleep.

If a few seconds under cold water makes you jump as if you've received a sudden jolt or energy boost, imagine what 10 or 15 minutes under a cold flow of water can do for you.

Here's how to energize yourself using cold water:

1. Let the cold water run while you get ready to take a shower.

2. Instead of "testing" the water temperature with your big toe, just get in there and let it run on both your hands and splash a small quantity onto your face. The water will not only hit your face but also a part of your torso, which will, in turn, make it easier for you to resist the cold temperature.

3. Now get completely under the shower head (repeating step 2). You might react to the cold water at first (it's never a pleasant thing), but your body will quickly adapt to it, allowing you to get used to the temperature as though you were numb to the cold.

4. Turn around and make sure your back is also exposed to the cold water. You will start to feel more energized during this phase of the cold shower (since your body is really getting the blood flowing to warm you up).

The goal is to maintain this reaction (body warming up due to the cold water) for long so that all your senses are revitalized.

This type of energizing session is ideal in the morning when you are ready to go to work, or even after a workout session, where you need your energy to be renewed so that you can still get things done during the day. Basically, you can do this whenever you are feeling fatigue, laziness, or lack of motivation.

(Tip: If you're affected by the afternoon slump at work and can't take a cold shower, splash some icy cold water on your face instead as a quick, convenient alternative.)

ASSIGNMENT: Try this cold session in the morning before you start your day. Let the cold water run over your body for about 5 minutes, to really get a complete energy boost to start the day, or revitalization when you need it during the day.

HACK #2:

Apply Acupressure Points

Acupressure was first developed and used in traditional Chinese medicine. Practitioners believe that the body's vital energy (called "qi") flows along channels (invisible ones) also known as "meridians." It is when these channels are blocked that a person begins to experience pain or fatigue.

When it comes to energy, five vital points are recommended to manipulate and encourage blood flow and energy flow by pressing on them with your thumbs or middle fingers. The purpose of pressing on these points is to bring an instant energy flow into the body by releasing natural painkillers (also called "endorphins"), which are very effective for people struggling with insomnia and fatigue.

This is how you should proceed here:

1. Place your thumbs at the base of your skull and press firmly (applying pressure), while slowly massaging from left to right and then from right to left. Apply the pressure and continue to massage for 3 minutes.

2. Move on to your second point, which is the pad between the joint of your thumb and your index finger. Here, again, apply some pressure and rotate using your fingers from left to right and then right to left, slowly for 3 minutes. Repeat the same thing with your other hand.

3. Your third spot will be the soles of each of your feet, at about one-third of the distance from your toes. Massage the whole area by pressing on it the same way you've proceeded previously, very slowly. Do the same thing with both feet, and remember to continue applying pressure for 3 minutes per foot.

4. Now comes the massage of the top center of your head. Press firmly with both hands, your thumbs at the back and middle fingers ahead. Press and rotate your fingers from left to right and right to left for 3 minutes. Here again, make sure your motions are slow and gentle on your head.

5. Your last point of pressure will be applied to the outside of your leg, at about 3 inches down from the kneecap. This time use your thumbs and middle fingers and operate in this area for 3 minutes on each leg.

Remember to proceed with the massage very slowly and press firmly but not too hard on each body part. It will take at most 30 minutes (or less), and you will feel completely revitalized after this. Apply this technique at least once a week to really feel its effects, and take advantage of it every day.

ASSIGNMENT: Practice this massage technique on the body parts mentioned. Remember that for the pressure to be effective, you will mostly use your thumbs and sometimes your middle fingers. Move slowly and from left to right and then right to left for 3 minutes on each body part.

HACK #3:

Breathe New Life into Body

There's nothing better than breathing in and out mindfully and letting fresh air into your body.

Fitness lovers of many kinds and coaches often encourage this practice of deep breathing during or after a workout because they know all too well the benefits of breathing.

For instance, during a yoga class, you will be instructed through several breathing sessions that will provide a healing pause or even complete the class. Coaches often ask their clients to take big breaths, for no other reason than simply revitalizing the body at crucial intervals with oxygen.

So here's how to breathe effectively to boost your energy:

1. Close your eyes to concentrate more fully on breathing. You might be stressed out, unmotivated, or simply tired when you do this. Closing your eyes helps to shut out those feelings and distractions, so that you can begin to leave point A (your state of tiredness and exhaustion) for point B (a state of vital energy).

2. Lift your arms a little bit and exhale, imagining that you are exhaling all the fatigue and lack of motivation from your lungs, your legs, arms and fingertips, etc.

3. Inhale to bring in new fresh air, then exhale slowly to achieve the same goal as in step 2. (As you inhale, concentrate on inflating your diaphragm or lower abdomen; and when you exhale, deflate your diaphragm.)

4. Repeat steps 2 and 3 five times to renew the energy inside of you.

5. End the breathing session by breathing normally for 10 seconds. Start moving your fingers and toes when you reach ten. Rotate your neck from left to right 3 times, and do the same in the opposite direction 3 more times.

After this last step, open your eyes and enjoy the rest of your day. This should be practiced regularly, and can be done anywhere. It will only take short periods of time (from 5 to 10 minutes), and you will always feel the difference after completing a session.

ASSIGNMENT: Attempt this type of breathing right away and remember to close your eyes, mentally expelling all the negative emotion and exhaustion from your body by slowly and fully exhaling everything in your lungs. This will be a cleansing process. End the session by readopting a normal breathing rhythm for 10 seconds, then revive your toes, fingers, and your neck by moving them by the end of the session.

HACK #4:

Intake Vitamin C for a Boost

Drink natural orange juice every day because its high vitamin C content will help you absorb certain nutrients more efficiently and also help you fight fatigue.

As may have guessed, this tip is about savoring your orange juice, but not as you usually do it. The main objective here is to give your body an instant boost during those times when you feel exhausted.

1. Pour yourself a full serving of orange juice in a small glass, being sure to shake the bottle well first to ensure the pulp mixes well with the juice.

2. Take a sip and hold the juice in your mouth for 5 seconds, and you will feel a sensory explosion in your mouth (an explosion of sweetness, bitterness, and pulp).

3. Then swallow, and take a deep breath.

4. Take two more consecutive sips, where you will experience the same "boom" effect as in step 2.

5. Once you reach the last sip, swallow the orange juice with an aaaaah! (This will awaken your senses a bit more and give you that boost you've been looking for.)

This way of experiencing orange juice is like pushing all your senses to acknowledge the nutrients and flavor in the juice, thus making you more alert and more able to receive its benefits.

ASSIGNMENT: Whether you need a little energy boost in the morning or during the day, take small sips of orange juice and keep them in your mouth for 5 seconds, and then feel the explosion of flavor and nutrients going from your mouth to your head, and the rest of your body. End your last sip with a big aaaaah! And move on with your day.

HACK #5:

Massage Scalp to Relieve Tension

Another way to "revive your senses" during the day and make you feel fresh again is to massage your most important asset, which is your head.

Sometimes when you are exhausted and low on motivation, you need to relax the nerves on your head, especially the ones on top of the back of your scalp. It will work like sending electrical pulses from your fingers to your scalp in just a few seconds.

Now, let's begin:

1. Place your middle fingers on top of your scalp and start pressing smoothly, until you feel a warm sensation on the spot you are working on. This warm sensation

will send healthy signals to your brain, making it immediately more alert.

2. Go down to neck level, still massaging your scalp, until you feel a warm sensation on your scalp. Do the same on the sides. To keep your focus, close your eyes and enjoy the session.

3. Renew the massage session 3 times, always going from the middle to the back and then the front and sides of your scalp.

4. During this session, you will feel a tingly sensation on your spine. Think of this as an awakening moment, where your body suddenly reacts to the massage on your scalp with the warm sensation it gives to your head.

ASSIGNMENT: Now it's time to give it a try. Use your middle fingers and work from the middle, to the back and front, then to the sides. Let the warmth that the massage creates take over you and make you feel revived and ready for the rest of the day.

HACK #6:

Take Power Naps

Sleeping is what we all need to help our body and mind get "back on top," but with today's hectic lifestyles, getting the much-needed 8-hours-a-night sleep is not always possible. On top of that, the stress we constantly feel can also give us frequent insomnia.

Fret not. There are a few things that can help you regain your energy during the daytime when you haven't had enough nighttime sleep. Take a couple of power naps during the day when allowed and when you are free, to renew your energy level and make the most of the rest of your workday.

This is how you should proceed:

1. Choose two periods of the day when you often feel you are low on energy (this is when you want to reboot your energy levels discreetly during the day, with a nap routine). It could be 10 minutes after lunch, or just around 11 a.m. before things get intense at work, or around 2:30 p.m. when you usually suffer from the afternoon slump. Pick two of these periods during the day, not more (as you may have a lot more work to do).

2. Use these two periods during the day to take some energizing power naps. Make sure you are freely situated with no interruption or distraction. Rest either lying comfortably on your back with some kind of support (in your car, with small pillows, cover, etc.) or on a flat surface where you can rest your head on your arms (such as with arms crossed on the table for comfortable head support).

3. Set your timer to 15 minutes for the first nap and 15 for the second nap. Completely let yourself go with these 15 minutes to becoming fully rested, and don't

worry about anything else. The timer will tell you when it's time to wake up. Being mentally prepared to let yourself go into a deep restoration period during these 15 minutes will help you take advantage of the nap and let you wake up feeling as though you've slept for maybe an hour longer than you have, rather than such short period.

That's the power of these power naps, and they can really help you during the day.

ASSIGNMENT: Now it's your turn to take some power naps and see the almost magical effect they have on your productivity. Remember, these are power naps, so they should be just naps to recharge your battery and not opportunities to slack off. Use a timer and jump right back to work straightaway after the nap is over.

HACK #7:

Experience the Sugar Rush

Do you know what they say about sugar when you ingest some while studying? From what we know, it has to do with the way it helps people regain their concentration.

Here's a neat hack that will allow you to regain a decent level of energy, using just a small amount of dark chocolate; or, if you're not the sweet-tooth type, you can opt for super-minty chewing gum instead.

1. Cut a square of the chocolate or take one piece of gum (if you prefer) and put it in your mouth. You will begin to feel the flavor of either the chocolate or the gum as a sign that your senses are engaged.

2. Start chewing on the chocolate or the gum. Their sugar content will give you an instant energy boost—all while the flavor (chocolate or mint) will have an effect on your senses of taste and smell, thus stimulating reactions that improve alertness.

3. After you swallow the first chocolate square or chew your gum to the point it's out of flavor, take another bite of chocolate or a second piece of gum. Take a few breaths and shake your head slightly from left to right (as a way to awaken yourself a bit more).

4. Optional: Chew on one more piece of chocolate or gum (which is supposed to seal the session), then proceed on with your day.

ASSIGNMENT: Try this technique right away with chocolate or gum (whichever you prefer), and send the right vibrations to your body in no time.

HACK #8:

Upgrade Energy Level with Superfoods

There's nothing better than turning to nature when we want to heal our body (without side effects). Our main problem, however, is that we either lack proper information or can't be bothered doing research about natural methods.

In other words (and not to be harsh), it's your loss if you haven't heard about the "superfoods" that can revive your energy. It's about time you grabbed one of them, like the incredible wheatgrass—a superfood that contains almost all the ingredients you'll need in order to maintain not only a healthy body but also the energy you need on a daily basis.

Its properties:

- One, it is known as an effective healer that contains many nutrients, including vitamins A, B (complex), C, E, I, and K.

- Two, it is rich in protein and 17 amino acids.

- Three, it contains 70% chlorophyll. The chlorophyll it contains is known as the first product of light and contains more light energy than any other food element.

- Four, it can be taken in many forms—including capsules, powders, pills, and tablets. Yet, most nutritionists agree that its most effective form is when it is raw and perhaps grown in your kitchen or in your backyard with your other plants.

- Five, other than drinking it as a solo concoction, you can also add it to your fruit-juice based drinks such as smoothies, or in other recipes of your choice.

How to prepare wheatgrass juice:

Get your wheatgrass (fresh) from a health food store or produce market near you. If you prefer, you can purchase your own wheatgrass seeds to grow them at home; follow the directions on the seeds package, as they are normally very easy to follow.

When ready to prepare your shot, cut a portion of wheatgrass. For 2 servings, get:

- 115 grams of wheatgrass
- 2 or 3 cups of water (preferably filtered)
- 1 lemon

1. Chop the wheatgrass to measure at least one half of a cup.

2. Put your chopped wheatgrass into a blender with the 2 or 3 cups of filtered water.

3. Blend the wheatgrass and water together at the highest speed.

4. Place a mesh strainer over a clean glass cup; make sure you line the strainer with cheesecloth.

5. Pour your wheatgrass mixture into the glass cup through the cheesecloth and strainer (so that in the end, you end up with liquid with no grass residue).

6. In order to get the most out of the mixture, use a wooden spatula and press on the remaining wheatgrass to extract the rest of the liquid.

7. Squeeze your lemon juice into the glass cup of wheatgrass juice, and serve.

Gulp it down fast (like you would drink a shot of any beverage served at a bar). The taste is not the most pleasant (basically, it does taste like grass), but when you think about all the benefits it has—hopefully it becomes an acquired taste.

ASSIGNMENT: Try to prepare a mixture of wheatgrass juice several times a week (3 or 4 times a week), and drink it before you start your day. To take it up a notch, grow some wheatgrass in your kitchen by planting their seeds (you won't believe how fast they grow) in order to have some that can be freshly cut several times a week.

HACK #9:

Choose Bright Fiery Colors for Energy

Colors are often used to describe a state of mind, or to represent an idea. The principle that color is connected to emotion is often used by interior decorators.

For example, a room painted in brown or gray feels calm, staid, traditional, and perhaps even dull. A white room feels clean, bright, modern, and maybe even sanitary, like a hospital room.

Now, think about the color red.

When you see red, you probably immediately think of something vivid: blood, life, romance, energy. Along these lines, if you're looking for an energy recharge, you might think about using a bright and very symbolic color, like red.

1. Start by picking out something visible in your environment that is completely red. It might be a vase, an image, or even a plain red painting. Place it close to you in such a way that you can fill your area of vision with red.

2. First thing every morning, spend time surrounding yourself with red, thinking about what it represents—life and vitality—and breathe in and out deeply, almost inhaling its redness. This color can remind you of other things you might associate with energy, like a juicy red tomato ripened under a hot sun that you can crush into the palm of your hand and release a warm strong aroma of tomato puree.

ASSIGNMENT: Use a red image or painting; place it somewhere where you will feel that you are showered with this energy color. As you let the color red leave its energizing impression on you, think about life, vitality, and all things associated with this color that come to mind.

HACK #10:

Substitute the Usual Cup of Joe

We've got nothing against coffee, but the thing with coffee is that its effects will wear off after a while. Regular coffee consumption, due to its high doses of caffeine, over time, can adversely affect the quality of your sleep, and thus sap your energy as quickly as it gave it to you.

You should know that tea is a good substitute. And the list of benefits is endless:

- It comes in many blends and gourmet flavors, especially when it comes to herbal varieties rather than standard black tea.

- You can drink more of it without getting the same caffeine buzz as coffee.

- Some teas (such as chamomile tea) can even help you relax and focus.

- It's delicious.

Some suggested teas to look for:

- <u>Ginseng tea</u>: Not only does it improve your digestion, it also boosts your immune system.

- <u>Green tea</u>: It is said to be good for the heart and helps you stay active all day.

- <u>Matcha tea</u>: It improves your mental alertness and clarity and works as a superb energy booster.

- <u>Black tea</u>: Black tea is said to help increase energy and help enhance blood flow to the brain and stimulate the heart.

Most teas are relatively low in caffeine, so you can indulge in tea as much as you want during the day.

ASSIGNMENT: From now on, pick the type of tea you want. Make sure you let it steep in hot water for from one to five minutes—depending on the type—and then indulge with or without sugar all day long.

HACK #11:

Feed Off Others' Contagious Energy

People often say that moods are contagious. Now whether you agree with this or not, wouldn't it be in your best interest to verify if that's the case for you—recharging yourself by feeding off other energetic people's energy?

You can either look to or think about another person who you know is normally full of energy.

You know ... that person who always seems to be smiling, the one you can hear laughing from miles away because that's simply who they are. The person who seems to animate everything and everyone they touch, with infectious laughter, affectionate looks, hilarious jokes, and positive energy.

If you don't know any real person like this, think of a fictional person whom you can admire and wish to be.

With that person topmost in your mind, do the following:

1. Try smiling the way that person does, seated or standing.

2. Throw your hands up like you're a little kid cheering because the bell just rang, signaling the end of the school day, and now it's play time.

3. Start doing a little victory dance, one step forward, two on each side, turn, and raise your hands again.

4. Again, raise your hands (closing your fists this time) and perhaps say a discreet "bingo." The "bingo" is supposed to seal the practice, meaning that you are now energized with more vitality. Then move on through your day, feeling just a little more focus and joy.

Doing this works like a car that has just been repaired and now needs to be driven and tested to be considered fully recovered from its mechanical difficulties.

If you're lacking mental energy, draw some inspirational attitude from others to help you repair your own body and mind.

ASSIGNMENT: From now on, practice this by watching those joie de vivre folks around you who are full of life. With them in mind, simulate their smile, raise your hands, do a victory dance (still thinking about how happy they always are), and then do the bingo move to seal your renewed energy.

HACK #12:

Enjoy an All-Natural Morning Energy Elixir

Here is a small secret that will have you looking full of energy and is extremely good for your health as well.

Have a cup of warm lemon water in the morning before you do anything else as a part of your daily routine.

Now, how do you prepare this mixture? It is quite simple:

1. Use a fresh-squeezed lemon to get two teaspoons of lemon juice.

2. Mix it with warm water in a glass or cup.

3. Let it rest for a few seconds and then drink.

If the taste seems a little too sour to you, think about what it is supposed to do for your body.

Lemon has many benefits, such as helping to prevent kidney stones, and can also give your metabolism a boost so that you can have more energy throughout the day. Think about what this mixture will help you achieve, including a healthier weight, more discipline, and, of course, much more energy to use and hopefully accomplish more tasks during the day.

ASSIGNMENT: This may not taste like a delicious fruit smoothie, but it is an energy elixir that will help you "shine" and outperform your peers every day. So, grab a few lemons or some lemon juice and administer a generous amount (2 teaspoons) of lemon juice in your water. Warm it up for 60 seconds and voila!

HACK #13:

Avoid Brain Fog by Anchoring Positive Past Experiences

People with no energy often suffer from what we call "brain fog" or a "brain fart," which does sound kind of silly, but really describes the zombified state we find ourselves in when we have no energy at all.

There's nothing better than simple mood enhancers, such as a pleasant smell, encountering a name that leads you back to a special thought, or even spotting a photograph that puts a smile on your face and instantly reminds you of how special your life has always been and that you should move on with it by being a bit more enthusiastic. (*"Come on, buddy, you can do it!"*)

This is what we call "anchoring." So, to effectively use your past experiences to be anchored as energy boosters, take a pause at least twice a day.

1. During these little mental breaks, name the first positive memory that comes to your mind, for instance one Sunday afternoon at the beach, and then let that memory take over your universe for 10 minutes (make sure you set your timer before you begin).

2. Let the memory flow in, and relive the moment in its entirety (until the timer lets you know that the time is up).

4. Take a huge breath in every time you revisit an intense anchored moment, which symbolizes relief from any tension or feeling of exhaustion, while at the same time absorbing the same positive energy you are visualizing.

3. As soon as you hear the alert from the alarm clock, breathe out and come out of the vision.

You've just absorbed energizing colors, smells, sensations—overall, the energies that made you very enthusiastic once. This is good enough to enhance your mood and your blood flow for the day.

<u>ASSIGNMENT</u>: Try this exercise by first recalling an anchored wonderful memory, then absorb all of those details that will energize you for the rest of the day.

HACK #14:

Stretch Face and Back Muscles Extensively

Many of us find our legs or arms feel a bit heavy and painful sometimes, but when your head and mind are affected by some kind of heaviness or malaise, it's even more difficult to start your day.

What you're experiencing might not necessarily be a huge headache, but simply tensed-up facial nerves that can affect the way you think and feel, energy-wise.

Now then, for those days where your head does not want to "align" with the rest of your body, you should simply stretch your face (more precisely your facial muscles).

1. Pull with your thumbs and middle fingers a few inches away from the corners of your eyes, gently pressing, and slide along the forehead. Apply this stretching technique 20 times.

2. Move down to your cheeks and pull the skin on the side (not too hard, but you should feel the gentle pressure on your skin being pulled away from the muscles in this area). Then release. Repeat the process 15 times.

3. Go further down in the neck area under the lower jaw, and massage the skin downwards, as if you were doing a face lift, but in the opposite direction (down the jaw). Repeat this movement 20 times, slowly and gently.

You will feel your skin, facial nerves, and muscles becoming a little bit tingly. This is a good sign, as this stretching exercise promotes blood flow and helps you feel relaxed, almost as if you were taking an extended rejuvenating break.

<u>ASSIGNMENT</u>: You should repeat the stretching exercises 5 times during the day. Remember that the key to having a successful facial stretch session is to pull your skin slowly without pulling or grabbing it too firmly.

HACK #15:

Start the Day with Sweet Music to the Ears

One thing that has been said about music is "it gives a soul to the universe." Pretty deep, huh? But, this is actually true, especially for certain types of music (the ones with great lyrics, or great rhythms).

For our intended purpose of boosting your energy, get a very mood-enhancing type of music (or *your* type of music) and play it in the morning just after you wake up, and let it guide you through your routine (brushing your teeth, making coffee, working out, maybe taking a shower, etc.). Then bring that music to the car, where you may sing or hum along, and let the vibes of the music and lyrics take over your thoughts.

This is what it might look like (more or less):

1. The alarm clock wakes you up. Normally, people still want to add 10 minutes of snooze to their sleep when relying solely on the alarm clock. What you can do is put on your favorite album, or set your favorite song to play on your phone to wake you up, early in the morning.

2. Get up and let the music energize you: walk, move, brush your teeth, and prepare your coffee following the rhythm of the song. So, if for instance, you choose to listen to Rachmaninov's Symphony No. 2 every morning, you might slide from left to right as if you were dancing the waltz (at the emperor's court). This is when the energy from the music takes over your body and mind, and you are consciously recharging your body.

3. Move on with the same music in the car (or on the bus, subway, bike, or however you commute), and hum along till you reach your destination (work, school, the store), where you will either have to be more discreet or be attentive to any kind of directive (from your boss or colleagues).

4. You can carry on with listening to this song during the day when you feel a little bit low in energy. This will automatically set you back to the initial energy level you had in the morning because your mind is conditioned to recognize the song or music piece as having energy-recharging virtues.

ASSIGNMENT: Now it's time for you to try this sort of mental anchoring and set your favorite song to wake you up and guide your morning routine while charging you with maximum energy. Dance and hum your way to work, school, or to wherever you wish to go.

INFO UNLOCKED:

Battery Fully Recharged

We work hard every day, and, regardless of what we do for a living, the fact is that we are always active.

For you to stop taking care of your daily work obligations all of a sudden could mean risking the loss of everything. A day or two away from your responsibilities might not hurt, but what about when you come back to reality?

A lot of things are expected from us. Life can be demanding. Hence, having the energy to keep up with everything is crucial these days.

The good news is that staying on top of your game, always feeling fresh and full of energy, may be a simple matter of following some easy habits you can do every day, such as taking cold showers frequently or giving yourself a few massages every day on strategic spots of your body.

Also, there are some surprising energy hacks you'll enjoy, such as savoring a little dark chocolate or letting your favorite music revive your senses and help you draw on its rhythms to keep you moving all day long.

It's all about trying out the energy-boosting hacks that work best for you, and tweaking and combining them catalytically to turn you into an unstoppable force of nature.

Begin living your life with more strength and more energy!

Energy Hacks

www.ingramcontent.com/pod-product-compliance
Lightning Source LLC
Chambersburg PA
CBHW050758240726

48654CB00008B/534